Let Patients Help!

Let Patients Help!

A "patient engagement" handbook –
how doctors, nurses, patients and caregivers
can partner for better care

"e-Patient Dave" deBronkart
with Daniel Z. Sands, MD, MPH

Introduction by Eric J. Topol, M.D.

CREATESPACE INDEPENDENT PUBLISHING PLATFORM

First edition, v1.0, April 15, 2013

Publisher: CreateSpace Independent Publishing Platform
www.CreateSpace.com

ISBN: 1466306493
ISBN-13: 978-1466306493

Contents

Part 2: Ten Ways to Let Patients Help

Part 3: Tip sheets: How To Be e-Patients and Empowering Providers
With Dr. Danny Sands

Epilog: The Road Ahead

About the Author

Appendix: Stop the denial.

Foreword

By George Alexander, longtime friend
and publisher of my first book, from the online journal
I kept during my cancer: *Laugh, Sing, and Eat Like a Pig*

I remember vividly how shocked I was when I learned that Dave deBronkart, who I had known for decades, had serious — probably terminal — kidney cancer. And then, how startled (and impressed) I was that he was letting those of us who were concerned about him follow the details of his treatment on his daily on-line journal at CaringBridge.org.

Those posts were remarkable for their honest, candid revelations about Dave's emotional turmoil. Yes, the clinical details were all there — the consultations about treatments, the X-rays, CTs and MRIs that confirmed the grim prognosis and the spread of the cancer. But it was Dave's openness about his emotions that moved me. Was he chronicling his last days on earth? It seemed likely. He couldn't know what was in store for him, and yet he shared it all with the rest of us.

And it quickly became clear that Dave was not going to be a passive patient. He collected whatever information he could find online about his condition and the possible treatments. He shared it with us, his readers, and discussed it with his doctors. In his journal, he wrote about everything he encountered in his journey into the world of medical care — the bad as well as the good.

His primary doctor and oncologist were available via email or the hospital's patient portal,[1] and Dave made full use of that for questions, appointment-setting, and referrals. Thanks to pioneering work at his hospital in the 1990s, he was also able to consult parts of his own medical records online. (Shouldn't that be available to all of us?) These electronic tools kept Dave informed, and greatly sped up his ability get answers and be engaged in his treatment.

And, importantly, his doctor recommended a good online patient community, where he got invaluable advice and emotional support from his patient peers.

In the end, Dave narrowly escaped death, saved by a treatment most patients never hear about, which happened to be effective for him (though it is not for the majority of patients who try it). It's a miracle that Dave is still among us, and Dave is not letting that miracle go to waste.

Out of that experience a new mission in life emerged, and a blog. Then "Patient Dave became "e-Patient Dave," determined to empower patients and change their relationship with medical professionals.

I hope you are reading this in good health. But as Dave says in his speeches, "Patient is not a third-person word – your time will come." When the time arrives (as it inevitably will) that a serious illness threatens you or a loved one, you can follow the trail that Dave has blazed and be an empowered patient, Working with your doctor to find the right treatment, choosing the right place to have it done, making use of online tools.

The best time to start – to develop your e-patient skills – is now, before a crisis. In this little book Dave will point the way; the rest is up to you.

---

[1] "Patient portal" is the term for a website you can visit to view parts of your medical record. In the Veterans Administration it's called MyHealtheVet, some hospitals have a portal called MyChart, and so on. Note that these are typically glimpses, *not* your whole record – more on that in this book.

Preface

A short recap of my cancer and recovery

"There's something in your lung."

My life changed with those words, spoken to me by Dr. Danny Sands around 9:02 a.m. on January 3, 2007. The day before I'd gotten a routine shoulder x-ray, and "incidentally," as they say in medicine, they stumbled on something else: a spot in my lung that shouldn't be there. The radiologist called Dr. Sands, who saw what the radiologist saw and spoke those words to me.

The spot turned out to be kidney cancer that was all through my body, with metastases everywhere from my thigh bone to my tongue and skull. I almost died but was saved by great doctors at Boston's Beth Israel Deaconess Medical Center. I got a treatment that usually doesn't work, but for me it did, and by July 23 – just 6½ months later – my treatment ended, and I'm all better. The whole story is in my first book, *Laugh, Sing, and Eat Like a Pig*, and is told in videos of my speeches at <u>ePatientDave.com/videos</u>.

Along the way I was treated by great surgeons, great oncologists, great nurses and nurse practitioners. Importantly, I did everything I could to help my cause – including joining with other patients online, to learn and to prepare for my treatment. Today, as described in this book, my oncologist says he doesn't know if I'd have survived if I hadn't been so involved.

As described in the Foreword, after my illness I found myself tumbling down an Alice's Wonderland rabbit hole, becoming "e-Patient Dave," blogging, suddenly testifying in Washington, and now giving speeches about how empowered, engaged, activated "e-patients" are changing what's possible in medicine.

But I've learned there's a problem – a big problem – and that's what this book is about. The problem is that **our culture assumes doctors know everything and patients can't possibly add anything useful.**

It's not just doctors who think that – most patients do, too.

Because of the cultural disconnect, most patients don't speak up. And when activated patients do, it's often sneered at, or politely dismissed with a "stay off the internet." (This isn't universal; some doctors and nurses "get it." But if you yourself haven't experienced being put in your place (at least gently), ask your friends and neighbors. I've never seen a case where stories of disrespect are more than one person away from any individual.)

A key challenge is that people who've had years of hard training and decades of experience have **good reason to wonder** what could possibly be added by people without that background.

It turns out the answer is, a lot can be added. But making it a reality takes work. So the question arises: "What could be said that would make any difference?"

My answer to that, which is happily gaining some acceptance, is the title of this book: Let Patients Help.[1]

---

[1] If you haven't seen it, the phrase comes from a chant I used at the end of a short speech I gave at a TEDx conference in Holland. The 16 minute video is at on.TED.com/Dave.

Acknowledgements

Wikipedia says this section is to be used to acknowledge people who helped during the writing of this book. Well, I want to use it to acknowledge some of the people without whom this book's message wouldn't exist – or without whom the world wouldn't be changing to make "let patients help" a practical possibility.

My problem is that there are so many, I know I'll leave some out. You'll know who you are, and you know me; you know you can hit me up so I'll include you next time. You know I'm grateful.

Early pals, out-of-the-nest pushers, and encouragers:
Susannah Fox, Alexandra Drane, Claudia Williams & husband David Witzel, Cindy Throop, Christine Kraft, Matthew Holt, Jane Sarasohn-Kahn, Jim Conway.

My very first speech-hirers: Gunther Eysenbach of Medicine 2.0 (first to ever offer me a keynote); Kent Bottles, then of ICSI (first to ever offer me a paying gig – arguably he kindled all that followed).

The first to ask me to attend a Washington policy meeting: Deven McGraw of the Center for Democracy & Technology, via her then-consultant Lygeia Ricciardi.

The health policy people in Washington who are working, and have worked, to bring computers FINALLY(!!) into American medicine, and to for HEAVEN'S sake let patients and families see their records. My challenge here is that I've personally worked with only a few of them, so I'll honor them all through these few: Chief Technical Officer Todd "Data Liberación!" Park; National Coordinators Rob Kolodner, David Blumenthal and (especially) Farzad Mostashari; Claudia Williams, Lygeia Ricciardi and teams.

You people are creating great new things for families across America. I personally thank you. Creating government policy in a trillions-of-dollars industry is a massive, difficult task, and implementing the policy is even harder. I salute your achievements.

Everyone who submitted corrections and suggestions.

For similar reasons I'm deeply moved by the **patients and advocates** who've worked so hard for so many years to bring the patient and family perspective to the national stage. There are too many to even start naming them, but I'll honor them all by citing one that touches millions of lives every year: **the National Partnership for Women and Families.** They're the creator of the Family and Medical Leave Act, which grants new parents the right to some time off at birth. That policy too was extremely hard, and "the Partnership" did it.

Finally, this book would surely not exist without the vision and execution of **Lucien Engelen** of the REshape & Innovation Center at Radboud University Medical Center in the Netherlands. Among Lucien's other accomplishments, these are relevant to this article:

- Creator and Curator of TEDxMaastricht, the 2011 event where my now-famous talk ended with the chant "Let Patients Help."
  - In announcing that event, he decided early on that the first announced speaker at this healthcare event would *not* be a ticket-drawing celebrity, it would be a patient. He announced this in April 2010!
  - His vision created the talk, the movement and the book.
  - That TEDx became the "Future of Health" conference series.

- Creator of the "Patients Included" badge that opens Part 2 of this book. Lucien "gets it" that the patient perspective *must be heard* if medicine is to improve successfully. "Patients Included" means he will no longer attend (nor speak at) any event where patient presence in the conversation isn't actively supported.

That's leadership – with integrity. Thanks to him, and to all of you.

Let Patients Help!

Introduction

By Eric J. Topol, M.D.

An extraordinary paradox exists in medicine and health care today. On the one hand, as a recent *Consumer Reports* cover article on cancer tests pointed out "cancer screening remains stuck in a 1960s view of the disease."[1] This problem of being stuck in our ways is much broader than cancer screening and can certainly be viewed to be operative across the board in health care. On the other hand, we have the newfound potential to obtain unparalleled, critical data and information about each individual. Whether this is via wearable sensors that capture one's vital signs or sequencing the DNA that comprises one's genome, we have new tools at our disposal – tools that were not available just a couple of years ago.

The buzzword of "big data" is used to refer to the immense amount of data that is currently being generated throughout the world — more than a zettabyte per year (that is 1,000,000,000,000,000,000,000 bytes). At the same time we can now generate "big data" for each individual and define his or her medical essence. So we have entered an unprecedented time of the information era finally invading and converging with the medical world.

---

[1] "Save Your Life: 3 Cancer Tests you Need Plus 8 You Don't." *Consumer Reports*, March 2013

Moreover, this information is flowing in a new way. Until now, doctors had full control of the data and information. We ordered the tests and scans and there was relatively little sharing of the results. Oftentimes patients have to contact a doctor repeatedly to get results of their laboratory tests or procedures. A marked asymmetry of access to the information has thus been characteristic.

But this is about to change. Now sensor data for key medical metrics like blood pressure, blood glucose, heart rhythm, and what seemingly is an endless list, can all be displayed on one's cell phone. That data can be automatically processed via software algorithms, whether built into the phone or via cloud computing in our wireless, hyper-connected world, to very useful information.

And now the information is directly available to the patient. A person's DNA sequence of six billion letters with all of the relevant annotation can be directly visualized on a tablet. These little mobile devices are the property of the individual, as should be the case for his or her data and information. In recent years the term "shared decision" has referred to the ideal scenario when the doctor and patient jointly discuss the choices and make an informed decision together. But now, with the emerging era of "information parity" there is a new "share" decision—will the patient even share the data with his doctor, or just make use of software processing?

In a recent article in *The New Yorker*, Michael Specter wrote "the era of paternalistic medicine, where the doctor knew best and the patient felt lucky to have him, has ended."[1] That is indeed true, and will become increasingly apparent in the near future. A new model of medicine is being induced by the digital era and the altered way in which information will be flowing.

For this and many other reasons, Dave deBronkart's new book is exceptionally timely. Instead of the old way of the authoritative doctor, we need to welcome and nurture a partnership model whereby each patient is fully engaged, informed, activated and intimately involved with his or her medical arc. Instead of the doctor

---

[1] Michael Specter, "The Operator," *The New Yorker*, February 4, 2013

Let Patients Help!

necessarily having sole access to one's data, taking on a look of exclusivity, it is time for each patient to take charge, to seize their own data. The term "empowered" doesn't do the concept justice. The mantra "Nothing about me without me" needs to rule the day.[1] To support this partnership in a world of information parity, the role of doctors can be transformed as the provider of advice, guidance, wisdom, experience, empathy, and communication.

As a survivor of what is usually a rapidly fatal kidney cancer, "e-Patient Dave" is widely considered one of the country's leading patient activists. His personal experience and willingness to share remarkable insights serves a basis for this guide. This book will unquestionably help many individuals become more active and fully engaged in their health care. Just what the patient ordered!

Eric J. Topol, MD
Author, *Creative Destruction of Medicine*
Professor of Genomics, The Scripps Research Institute
Cardiologist, Scripps Clinic

March 17, 2013
La Jolla, California

---

[1] Pauline Chen, Letting Patients Read the Doctor's Notes, *New York Times,* October 4, 2012.

Dedication

To my daughter Lindsey,
whose life has been my biggest bonus for surviving;

to her husband Jon,
her partner in the life I get to watch,

and to their baby girl being born this summer,
whose life-to-be brings me tears of joy.

It is for our future generations
that we're building a new and better world
of health, care, and medicine when we need it.

Nashua, New Hampshire
March 2013

Basics 1:
Roots of the Movement

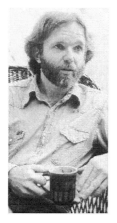

In medicine, a lot of your ability to do valuable things depends on how much you know. Few people understood this as well as "Doc Tom" Ferguson, founder of the e-patient movement.

In 1978 Tom graduated from Yale Medical School. He never practiced, but he published, with a strong emphasis on sharing his knowledge with patients, enabling them to do as much as they could for themselves and their families.

He became medical editor of the *Whole Earth Catalog,* whose subtitle was "Access to Tools." He published *Medical Self-Care* magazine, and a book of the same name. He appeared on *The Today Show* and *60 Minutes,* and in John Naisbitt's landmark 1982 book *Megatrends.*

Ferguson knew we could do a lot for our families, but he also knew our abilities were limited by access to information. And when the internet came along, that changed everything. His friends say that as he observed what people could newly do, he wondered what to call this new kind of connected patient. Eventually, they say, he settled on "e-patient."

Initially, they say, the e was for electronic. As time went by, other meanings were invented: empowered, engaged, equipped, enabled. Today some add educated, expert, and anything else e.

Doc Tom had multiple myeloma, and died unexpectedly in 2006 while hospitalized for a relatively routine treatment. He was in the middle of researching and writing a substantial report for the Robert Wood Johnson Foundation's Pioneer Portfolio, where they like to study the fringes of healthcare, to better understand what the future might hold.

The paper was about this new type of patient, and was titled "e-patients: how they can help us heal health care." After his death his colleagues finished it, and today you can download it free, in English or Spanish, from e-patients.net, the blog Tom started.

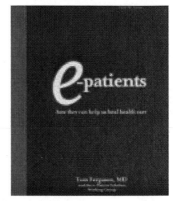

In 2009 a number of Tom's followers decided the time had come to formalize the work, and incorporated as the Society for Participatory Medicine, which lives today at ParticipatoryMedicine.org.

Recognizing the importance of the network aspect of Tom's vision, and the new kind of partnership Doc Tom envisioned, they defined participatory medicine as:

> A movement in which networked patients shift from being mere passengers to responsible drivers of their health, and in which providers welcome and value them as full partners.

Among Tom's followers was Dr. Danny Sands, who was my primary physician when my cancer struck. Putting their money where their mouth is, they said this society can't be run by a doctor alone – it's about partnerships. And they elected Dr. Sands and me as co-chairs for the first few years. Yeah, a patient as a co-chair of a medical society. How crazy is that?

Or is it? Can patients help heal healthcare?

Let Patients Help!

Basics 2:
What Empowered
and Engaged mean
(and a short glossary)

Empowered

An empowered person knows what she wants[1]
and speaks up.

A disempowered person,
faced with a challenge, will say,
"There's nothin' *I* can do about it."
That's the hallmark of being powerless.

Facing the same challenge, **an empowered person**
thinks "What *can* I do?" ... no matter what the odds.

Engaged

To be engaged is to be involved, active, responding.

An engaged patient listens, responds,
asks questions, thinks for herself, and acts.

A disengaged patient treats healthcare like a carwash:
rolls up the windows, sits back and gets things sprayed on him.

---

[1] In this book genders are mixed at random.

A Short Glossary (read this!)
for those new to medicine

The culture of medicine is changing, as we change our beliefs about who's supposed to do what and who's capable of what. And when culture changes, people sometimes get upset, because Person A says something in the new view and Person B hears it in the old, or vice versa, and if they don't realize meanings are changing, either party can think the other one is lying, insulting, or an idiot. The remedy is to be clear about meanings.

Here are definitions of a few insider terms that have useful meaning but which normal people find weird. If you have questions, post them as a comment at the bottom of epatientdave.com/books and maybe they'll go in the next edition.

"Patient Engagement"

This book is about what the industry calls "patient engagement." People mean many different things when they say this, and that's a setup for disconnect. To some people "patient engagement" is simply about whether you're taking your pills and buying more.[1] But as I said on the previous page: engaged patients are actively involved in all aspects of their care, and perhaps even in designing what care should be.

e-Patient:

A patient who's empowered, engaged, equipped, enabled – see "Roots of the Movement" a few pages back.

Types of people who work in the industry

*   **Clinicians**: trained medical professionals who work in clinics, hospitals, etc. Basically, doctors and nurses.

---

[1] Guess what business *those* observers are in.

Let Patients Help!

- **Providers**: people and businesses who provide medical services – generally clinicians and the places where they work.

- **Payers** is a term that drives me nuts because it's so centered around the *provider's* pocketbook. To most hospitals the bills are paid by **insurance companies**, so that's who they call payers. It's ironic because for the most part, insurers get *their* money from us – workers and employers. *We're* the ones who pay to get services.

Terms related to the changing role of the patient

- **Patient:** in this book, "patient" is the person receiving medical services because of a problem or a checkup. Often it also includes the patient's **caregivers:**

- **Caregivers** are the people (family or other, paid or not) who help care for a person who can't manage on their own. (Usually that person is a child, elder, or person with a condition that requires help.) Like the patient, the caregiver receives instructions and (we hope) helps carry them out.

- **Consumers,** in this book, also refers to the people who receive services, but **in a different context: as choosers and buyers of care.** Some people find "consumer" to be an empowering word ("one who gathers information and makes informed choices"), and others say it's belittling ("a pawn of the sell-sell-sell establishment"). I use the term when the context is business instead of medicine.

Terms related to who calls the shots

- **Paternalism** or paternalistic medicine: The paternalistic view says patients can't understand anything important so clinicians have to bear the responsibility. The term comes from the reality that parents need to take care of kids. Some patients want to be treated that way (fine with me), but empowered/engaged patients want to be partners – exactly as if they were children who've grown up, learned to think for themselves, and are ready to share responsibility.

- **Compliance** or **adherence**: This term is a direct outgrowth of paternalistic thinking, though clinicians often don't realize it. It's whether or not you do as you're told: the provider prescribes (medications or treatments), and if you do it, you're "compliant." It's an obnoxious belittling word, so some providers soften it to "adherent." But that's still focused on whether you're doing what *they* told you to.

My view: patients are the ultimate stakeholders – the ones who live or die, suffer or improve, based on how it all works out. In my view, treatment goals should arise in discussion between clinicians and patients. And if *I'm* the one who sets the *goal* of the treatment, I call it **achievement,** not behaving myself!

Which is more inspiring to you?

With that understood, let's get on with it. What follows is what I've learned from participating in two hundred meetings about health and medicine since this "e-Patient Dave" thing happened. It's not just my opinion for its own sake; the items in these pages are things others have said shed new light on the future of medicine – for them.

Part 1:

Ten Fundamental Truths about Health and Care

"A book can save your life."

*- An e-patient whose wife believes she was saved
after she learned about patient communities
and found three that helped her treatment*

1.

Patient is not a third person word

The first health event I ever spoke at was a half-day panel at the Hyatt Regency in Cambridge, MA. It had brilliant symbolism: for the first half of the day they left one seat empty – the patient's. After the break they brought me up.

As the panel progressed, I was the last to speak. (I was glad, having never attended any such meeting.) Without any forethought, these were the first words out of my mouth:

> I want to propose that we modify our language. We're all talking about patients as if they're someone who's not in the room – someone out there on the street.

> Well, I'm here to tell you, **patient is not a third person word.** Whether it's you yourself, your child, your spouse, your mother – **your time will come**, when *you're* the one in the hospital bed, or *you're* the one at the bedside, holding someone's hand and silently thinking, "Dear God, I hope she makes it."

Trust me, whether it's this year or next year or ten years from now, what happened to me is coming to your breakfast table. So as you think about all the issues in this book and in medicine, think of it that way.

The problem is, it's hard to do that until you're actually in the crucible. As my friend Perry, who has Parkinson's, says: "Until your days are numbered, you don't *know* what's important."

Do your best to absorb this before the stuff hits the fan for your family.

2.

Patients are the most under-used resource

Warner Slack is a senior physician at my hospital, Beth Israel Deaconess Medical Center in Boston. A wise and wonderful man, he's been saying since the 1970s that patients are the most under-used resource.

Originally he said "the most under-used resource in our information systems," saying patients could do a lot of the data entry into an electronic medical record. How visionary is that? **Forty years later** we're getting to a version of that view – patient engagement with the medical record. It took an act of Congress and years of hearings to write the regulations requiring it. Listen to Warner, people![1]

Today many of us quote him on this, and paraphrase it: the most under-used resource in health [and] care, or the most under-used member of the healthcare team. Any patient or family member who's been disregarded by professionals knows how under-used we can be.

Why is this, you ask? My guess is that it's an assumption woven into our culture: trained medical professionals can do things nobody else can (true), so *nobody else could possibly contribute anything* (false).

---

[1] Happily for me, long ago Dr. Slack mentored my primary physician, Dr. Danny Sands.

We can transform this: culture is a set of persisting conversations about what's possible and what's appropriate. New conversation: Let Patients Help.

3.

We all know something.
No one knows everything.
(Not even doctors.)

This one's tricky, because it interferes with our instinctive desire to find a genius who knows everything: someone who knows exactly what's wrong with us (or our baby), and exactly what to do.

I felt it myself when I was sick: I absolutely wanted to feel that I was in the best place in the world, and that my physicians would do everything in their power to scour the earth for every possible option, and use their years of training and experience to make the perfect decision.

But it's not possible: there's too much for anyone to know everything, even *your* doctor. And if you and s/he both act like knowing everything is possible, it's a setup for dysfunction: any shortfall seems like a betrayal.

Here's reality:

- There were 800,000 new articles published in medical journals in 2010 alone, and the number keeps going up.

- Paul Grundy MD, IBM's director of worldwide healthcare transformation, told me the average primary care doctor has

1500-2000 patients. Imagine how many conditions s/he has to keep up on.[1]

- My own oncologist, Dr. David McDermott, says it's true: "Unless you're a sub-sub-specialist like me, it's impossible to keep up."

A growing number of clinicians understand this, but many don't, and get defensive: "You can't possibly know everything" seems so anti-establishment, so disrespectful. So I went to an authority. In Doc Tom's white paper he quotes Dr. Donald Lindberg, director of the National Library of Medicine:

> If I read and memorized two medical journal articles every night, by the end of a year I'd be 400 years behind.[2]

When I started giving speeches I'd quote him at conferences, thinking he'd be enough of an authority. But doctors would *still* come up and say they doubted it. So in 2010 when I spoke at "the Library" and met Dr. Lindberg, I asked him if it's still true. His response? "Oh, it's much worse."

Clinicians have information overload, but the internet lets ordinary patients see information that their doctors might not. Yikes: does *that* clash with our cultural assumption!

Lesson, for patients and clinicians:

- Anyone whose sense of self-worth depends on knowing everything is in big trouble.

- It's no failure on anyone's part if a less trained person has seen something they haven't.

- But there's still no substitute for *the trained mind*, with years of clinical experience, to put it all in perspective.

Let Patients Help.

---

[1] I recently heard there's a list of 11,000 conditions, but I haven't found the source.
[2] Page 34

4.

Googling is a sign
of patient engagement

In my high school days
(in the time of Noah's Ark)
there was a funky dance
called the bugaloo.[1] Today
it's back, in a different form
I call the e-Patient Boogloo:
searching for health
information on Bing,
Google and Yahoo.

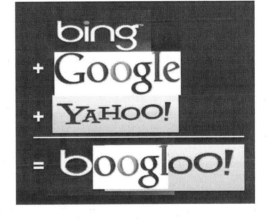

It's America's most popular
way of engaging in our
health. A good thing, right?
But when patients bring these ideas to their doctor, often I'm told the
doc's eyes roll and they're told, "Stay off the internet."

The truth: it's often said there are more searches every day for health
information in America than there are doctor visits. Susannah Fox at
the Pew Internet and American Life project reports:[2]

---

[1] Years later there was a different version; look it up on YouTube.
[2] For more data from Susannah and her colleagues visit
bit.ly/PewHealthTips. It's updated whenever new research is done.

- 81% of US adults use the internet
- 72% of them have sought health information in the past year.

Do the math: 81% x 72% = 58% of US adults have searched for health information in the past year. And that's increasing as the younger become older, and "digital natives" become adults.

"Naa," you say, "my patients aren't like that." Well, perhaps not the patient herself – but Pew data says half of health searches are for someone else. I call it **e-Patient by Proxy.**

I'm not saying everything people find is gold; there certainly is crap on the internet. That's why in my vision of the medical home of the future, one role will be **Information Coach** – someone to whom you can say, "I found this site – what do you think?" Teaching people to evaluate sites will put competence in the home, where it belongs. In the hands of citizen patients.[1]

If patients don't know how to do the "Boogloo" safely, don't stop them from engaging – teach them how. Or, as I said in my 2010 testimony to a workgroup creating new regulations for electronic medical records:

Until people gain experience,
they're inexperienced!

The solution is not to restrict and constrain.
Empower the people: enable, and train.

---

[1] In Part 3 of this book my primary physician, Dr. Danny Sands, provides his advice on good web use.

5.

We perform better
when we're informed better

Nobody can do their best if they don't have relevant facts. This has turned out to be one of the most pervasive cultural disconnects I've seen in medicine: we expect people to do a great job, even if they don't have the information they need.

It applies to patients:

- They can't understand a disease or treatment if they can't find information on it.
- They can't understand their status – and react – if we hide the data from them.
- They can't follow instructions if they're not written clearly.
- They can't control costs if we hide costs from them.

Perversely, problems like this are commonly described as health *literacy* problems. Too often it's health *clarity* problems. Before we insult a learner let's try to make it clearer.

But it applies just as forcefully to the professionals who care for patients. **No clinician can possibly perform to the top of their training** if they don't have relevant facts:

- They can't recommend the best treatment if they don't *know* all the options. Including ones developed since they were in school.

- They can't respond to patients' needs if patients don't express them. (That would be you, patients. Speak up!)
- They can't diagnose smartly, or prescribe safely, if important information is missing (or wrong) in the chart.

Think about it: before a professional receives his license, he takes a license exam. You wouldn't expect a correct answer if some facts were withheld, right? Yet too often they're expected to perform *with live human subjects* when the information they're given is incomplete or poorly organized. That's not fair to them.

Remedies for providers – and their patients:

- **Offer patients information they can understand and use.**
  - o Take time to find out whether they understand it.
  - o Patients, *say* whether you understand it. Ask yourself, "Will I be able to explain this to the people who help me?" If not, you're not ready to be responsible and effective.

- **Let patients check the entire medical record,** then *fix any mistakes the patients find*. Otherwise, the next clinician will be given wrong instructions.
  - o Patients and caregivers, ask to check for errors in the record. If they say no, push back – it's *your* health that's at stake, not theirs. This is not a matter of what's convenient for them (or their "office policy.") Stick up for the person whose life is at stake.

You can't fault anyone – employee or patient – for not using information that they don't have, or can't understand.[1]

---

[1] If you *really* want to have fun, print some stickers that say THIS ISN'T CLEAR and let people put them anywhere they want. And assign someone to tally those, and fix 'em!

Let Patients Help!

6.

But information alone doesn't change behavior

We perform better when we're informed better – but that's not enough. If information alone were enough to create change, all we'd need is pamphlets.

Yet in conference after conference I see speaker after speaker who seems to think, "If we just hammer hard enough on the undeniable facts, things will change. If it's not working yet, give 'em more facts."

Wrong.

It doesn't work for diet and exercise. It doesn't work for getting people to take their medications. It doesn't work for getting clinicians to wash their hands. It doesn't work for preventing medical errors.

Behavior change is not rational. Find methods that work.

An epiphany for me was Daniel Kahneman's massive book *Thinking, Fast and Slow*[1] about "behavioral economics" – the study of why and how people perceive choices, and why and how they *make* a choice. **It's not rational** – *even when smart people have the information.* **Information alone doesn't change behavior. Even for smart people.**

---

[1] Kahneman, D. (2011). *Thinking, Fast and Slow*. New York: Farrar, Straus and Giroux.

A simpler, less weighty view of behavioral economics is in *Switch: How to Change Things When Change is Hard* by Chip and Dan Heath. It's widely cited for its "elephant, rider, and path" metaphor: the image is a rider on an elephant, following a path in a jungle:

- **The elephant** has all the power – the force. (The elephant is like our emotions and feelings.)

- **The rider** may be a great thinker, but if the elephant doesn't want to go where the rider says, guess who wins? (The rider is our intellect – rational thought.)

- **The path** is the surroundings, the environment. The elephant may be capable of bulling its way through the brush, but it's much easier to follow the path – the route that's convenient and points *mostly* in the right direction. Or not: the path is the path.

For us "the path" shows up in the many things that shape what's convenient in life. If there's no good food where you live, you're not likely to eat well. If it's hard to get to the doctor, you're not likely to go. If it's hard for someone to remember to take their pills, they don't. *Even when they know it's important.*

Stop trying to solve that by giving people more facts. A new approach is being tried now, based on behavioral economics: **Make it easier to do the right thing.** For instance, if your pill bottle has a GlowCap®, it reminds you when it's time – by glowing, beeping, or calling someone's phone. Amazingly (not), in early tests "compliance" boomed from 71% to 98%.

See what a mistake it is to think of it as the patient's failure?

Whether you're a patient, caregiver or provider, if something important is hard for a patient to do, speak up. And innovators, look for ways to make a killin' in the market by inventing things that *are* easier to do. The door's wide open, and boy do e-patients want it.

Because, you see …

7.

Clarity is power

In any other business, if your stuff's hard to use, you're out of business. Vendors learn to be clear or die. Similarly, when we find something medical is hard to understand, we should think like a company whose survival is at stake, and make it easier.

I know this first-hand. I once worked for a company developing two powerful typesetting systems. Both were confusing to our test users, and two statements from developers still ring in my mind:

> "It's perfectly clear once you understand it."
> (Someone responded, "Um, that's also true for nuclear physics.")

Then this, about a different product, at a board meeting:

> "Marketing isn't finding customers who are smart enough."

How'd that work out? Well, when typesetting was attacked by desktop publishing, our company was one of the first to die. *People liked the competitor better.*

There's more to the value of information than the information itself. Just as a medication is no good if it can't be absorbed, information is useless if it can't be absorbed. **Investing in clarity is just as important** as developing the facts and tools in the first place.

Examples:

- Thomas Goetz, then *Wired*'s executive editor, realized that his blood test results were incomprehensible rows of numbers. He asked his art directors to make them look like an investment report. They came back with snazzy, easy-to-read graphics: a bar for each number, green at the good end, red at the bad end, and an arrow showing where he sits. Bam: the same data, presented with better software, and the same slacker "consumer" suddenly becomes capable. Magic!

- Health Literacy Missouri is producing great results by translating medical speak into simpler language. (It was a visit to them in 2011 that led me to blog, "Clarity is power.")

- In the February 2013 issue of the *Health Affairs* policy journal there was an article about health *literacy* – but you know what it talked about? Improving the *clarity* of what we *give* the supposedly-not-literate-enough patients. Excellent! (But why do they still call it "literacy"?? Because the cultural assumption is that providers know things, and everyone else should understand but isn't "literate" enough.)

If you think patients and families need to be smarter, I encourage you to remember my colleagues in typesetting who said customers should be smarter. Please focus on what works: clarity.

As consumerism and customer choice come to medicine, any provider who wants to survive will be well advised to stop thinking like the product developers who said customers aren't smart enough. If what you want people to do is not easy for them to understand, make it easy.

8.

Health is not medicine.
Treatment is not care

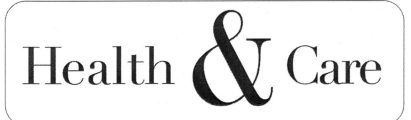

From a December 2012 blog post:

From now on for me it's not "healthcare," it's "health *and* care."

Why? Because I'm increasingly seeing that it's incomplete to look at transforming medicine by just talking about the care part – the part that kicks in when something goes wrong. All of us – patients and providers and insurance and government and industry and everyone – need to be thinking about health, every time we approach a problem with the health *care* system.

I know I'm not the first to say this, but as a marketing slogans guy ("Let Patients Help," "gimme my damn data" etc.), I'm keenly aware of the power of handy language. Everything I explained above can be said over and over, but it doesn't fit easily into everyday discourse. **"Health and care" is an easy plug-in replacement for the**

usual phrase "health care." And that boosts the odds people will use the new wording.

I say:

- The industry we call "healthcare" is mostly medicine, medical skills, and medical services. I love the industry for saving my life, but I call medicine medicine.

- Health is your health, your well-being. You can have plenty of health so you never need care. But I still prefer to get checkups – remember, I was saved by a discovery during a routine physical.

- Treatments are good, but they're separate from care. I know plenty of people who've gotten treatments with no care, and vice versa.

Language defines our thinking, so I say it's good to be clear about what we're discussing. Let's say medicine when we mean that, treatments when we mean that, and care when we mean care.

9.

The urge to care
for our families is strong

In high tech you learn to watch for why things take off. Some ideas set the world on fire, and others (just as sexy) don't. It's hard to predict – when the iPad was new, some blog posts said "Why can't Apple do anything right anymore?" It's hard.

So in my advocacy for patient engagement I've watched to see when there's resistance and when there's not, and it comes down to this:

> A lot of people aren't sure whether an adult like me really needs to nose around in his medical record. But nobody pushes back on a parent with a sick kid, or an adult caring for an elder at home.

When I realized that, I stopped talking just about patients and switched to "patients and families." A lot of the work of health and care is indeed *between* family members, not just self-care.

We also need to activate patients and families, get them thinking, asking questions, involved in health and care. There too, it seems easier to teach an adult to get involved in *another* person's care – their child, or their elder. I suspect we may find success if we teach adults their e-patient skills while they're caring for another. Then, perhaps those skills will be familiar when their own time comes.

"My mother-of-a-patient voice"

Kelly Young, the famous "RA Warrior,"[1] says she never had trouble being alert and assertive with her kids' pediatricians. Then, she says, she learned "to use my mother-of-a-patient voice" when talking to her own doctors. I love it.

See if you can think of yourself as being just as important as a child you care for, and just as worthy of effort and involvement.

---

[1] See her incredibly informative blog at RAWarrior.com, and the Rheumatoid Patient Foundation she started. *That's* one heck of an engaged, empowered patient – enabled by learning to use her mother-of-a-patient voice, to speak up for herself as she does for her kids.

10.

Patients know
what patients want to know

As someone whose life was saved by great medicine and great clinicians, I know there's life-saving value in the best that medical science has to offer. But it's not the only value.

There's life-saving value in knowing the biology of a tumor, a virus, a bacteria. But there's value, too, in practical facts you'll never see in a peer reviewed scientific journal, but you will find in patient communities. Why? Because scientists have their priorities, and patients have theirs. In my own case, within two hours of joining a patient community I heard this:

- Kidney cancer is an uncommon disease. Get yourself to a specialist center that does a lot of cases.

- There's no cure, but there's one treatment that usually has no effect but sometimes does, and when it does, about half the time it's complete and permanent.

- Most hospitals don't offer it, so you may not even be told it exists.

- The side effects are severe – they sometimes kill the patient. That's why you need a specialist center.

- Here are the names and phone numbers of four doctors near you who do it.

Clearly this is of value to patients, but *to this day, there's not a single peer-reviewed scientific resource that says it.* Why? Because scientists' priorities are valid, but patients need other information too.

Then when my time for treatment neared, I wanted to understand what to expect from those horrible side effects. No scientist's site helped, but my patient community sent me fifteen first-hand stories. No one of them would pass muster in a scientific journal, but they were all useful.

And here's the punch line: today my oncologist, Dr. David McDermott, says "I'm not sure you could have tolerated enough medicine if you hadn't been so well prepared."

There's life-saving value in medical science, but it's not all there is. Let Patients Help.

How? Read on.

Part 2:

Ten Ways to Let Patients Help

First hint:
To avoid mistakes caused by paternalistic thinking,
include patients in all planning, decisions,
conferences, and work teams.

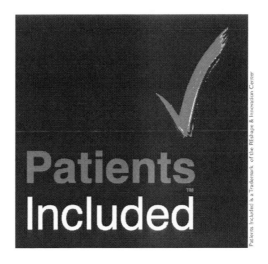

This "Patients Included" badge was conceived by my Dutch buddy
Lucien Engelen of the REshape & Innovation Center
at Radboud University Nijmegen Medical Centre,
Nijmegen, Netherlands.

1.

Let patients help:
give us our data!

For strange reasons, my first medical keynote was titled "Gimme My Damn Data."[1] To my amazement it went viral, spreading all over the internet, with thousands of web references, a coffee mug,[2] a rap,[3] and a rock song.[4]

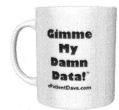

Why all the attention? Because a lot of patients want their data – *all* their data – and a lot of providers and computer system makers say there's no need for that. We disagree:

- Whose data is it?

- Who has more to gain (or lose) from the data being complete, accurate, and *available where it's needed*?

- Who has a right to limit what I might want to do with it?

At the simplest level, we want access to the chart – all the stuff the docs and nurses see. As Dr. Sands says, "How can patients participate if they can't see what I see?"

---

[1] Video of that lecture is at epatientdave.com/videos#med20

[2] bit.ly/datamug

[3] on.TED.com/Dave, at 12:00

[4] bit.ly/DataSong

Ask for Open Notes: In the U.S., new regulations will make access to our records a reality. A huge 2012 study called OpenNotes established that **it doesn't ruin doctors' lives.** And patients love it.

OpenNotes was a year-long study in three medical centers, funded by the Robert Wood Johnson Foundation. Patients were given unrestricted access to their physician's actual notes, in unaltered doctor-speak. Not only did patients love it (99% wanted to continue); many other benefits were reported, and 85-89% of patients said it would affect which providers they choose![1]

That's an early but potent sign of consumerism coming to medicine: **patient access is now a competitive business issue.** Patients, ask for access; providers, get ready. The evidence says *it doesn't hurt.*

At conferences I hear a lot of complaints about the idea of access, all boiling down to this: **"Patients don't understand this stuff."** And indeed, if you've never let someone see something, they won't understand it (yet). My view:

> ### It's perverse to keep people in the dark then call them ignorant.

Search these terms (in boldface) – they're early signs of real change, whose potential is clear:

- **"Blue Button+"** for medical records: The original "Blue Button" on some sites would let you *download* your medical data. The new "Blue Button+" will let you *connect* apps to your medical record.

- **Dr. Eric Topol,** who wrote the introduction to this book, is the guru of personal health gadgets – and what their data can do for us. Search for his TED talk "The wireless future of medicine."

- My buddy **Hugo Campos**, who has a defibrillator implanted in his heart. He wants access to *the raw data* coming out of his device … to help him stay well. The manufacturer says no!

---

[1] The evidence also said that contrary to fears, the study had hardly any impact on doctors' lives. So when the study ended, not a single doctor quit – not even the skeptics. Search "OpenNotes" to find the many articles and blog posts about this important study.

2.

Let patients help
take care of their families

The urge to take care of our families is strong. When a patient's in the hospital, *welcome* the family's desire to understand what's happening and participate in the patient's care.

- **Welcome patients' efforts to check the chart.** My friend Marge Benham-Hutchins talks of how she was always on top of her husband's lab results, etc., through the hospital's portal … until he became an in-patient, and then they wouldn't let her look! How silly is that?? Hospitalization is no time to *stop* patient engagement.

    o Some forward-thinking hospitals even **let families write in the chart.** Why not?? Provide a place for patient and family notes – and be sure the care team reads them.

- **Welcome questions.** It's not rude for patients (and families and caregivers) to ask questions – it's patient engagement! Be grateful. (Patients, ask away! Respect their time, but engage!)

- **Clinicians should change shifts[1] at the bedside,** so patient and family can listen as one shift gives report to the next. I'm told

---

[1] "Shift change" is when clinicians go off duty and hand off responsibility to the next shift, telling them each patient's status. It can be a busy time, and communication errors aren't rare – it really helps when family listens.

countless studies have shown this reduces communication errors, from medication changes to how the patient's doing. Think about it: every provider coming on shift depends on the chart being accurate, but nothing guarantees it will be – so how can they do a good job? Let patients help reduce errors.

- **Welcome family efforts to check for correct meds.** There's *nothing* in the modern hospital that insures perfection – let patients help.

- **Support family engagement, with comfortable overnight accommodations.** As great as my hospital was, we felt insulted at the horrible "recliners" they offered for my wife to spend the night. We had enough stress from the cancer; did they need to add sleep deprivation?

Why not share the care plan?

Too often we put all the burden on overworked clinicians, who don't work in a fail-safe system. Let patients help.

In his 2010 Stanford commencement address, famed surgeon and author Atul Gawande told of Duane Smith, who survived a horrible head-on crash. He lost his spleen but with spectacular treatment he was discharged weeks later in good condition – except they forgot to give him the three vaccines a splenectomy patient should get.

Two years later on vacation he picked up an infection and it raced through his body; again he recovered, but lost his fingers and toes.

What if his family had googled splenectomy, and said, "Wasn't he supposed to get some vaccines?" Or, what if the hospital had shared the care plan? Some hospitals do it[1] – why not yours?

---

[1] Abington Memorial, in Pennsylvania, prints a daily report from their medical record system, in layman's language, so family can follow along. They say it's not at all rare for patients to spot an oversight. Free quality improvement!

3.

Let patients help
scour the earth for information

When patients and family want to Boogloo, don't complain –
give lessons.

They might just be trying to understand – to be engaged and
informed! Or in a difficult case, they might be trying to find
something the doc hasn't seen. *This is no insult to the clinician.*
Let patients help.

Remember Dr. Lindberg: *nobody* can know everything anymore.
He said reading two articles a night would put him behind by 400:1.
Today it's worse – in 2010 alone over 800,000 articles were indexed
by the Medline publication system.

Both patients and clinicians need to realize **it's no insult** if a patient
has seen something a clinician hasn't. Cases in point:

- Most patients with my disease never hear about the treatment I
  got, even though it's the only possible cure. It's not really the
  doc's fault – the official cancer database is out of date! But the
  patient community on ACOR.org knows the latest.

- Metastatic breast cancer patient Judy Feder prolonged her life
  18 months by finding a researcher who was studying a biological
  marker that looked interesting. She brought it to her oncologist
  (note the collaboration) and said, "What do you think?" They

tried a few things, and she gained 18 more months watching her grandchildren grow up.

- Mike Spencer, husband of Monique Doyle Spencer, found a remedy online for a painful chemo side effect his wife Monique was having, called "hand-foot syndrome." A simple paste made of henna and lemon juice, it worked – but not a single medical journal has ever described it.

This is not to say that everything online is gold; there's garbage too. But it's a mistake to tell patients to stay offline.

Remember the TV series "House MD"? He was a crusty old sot, famed for saying "When did *you* go to medical school?" when the family had an idea. He was out of touch with reality, in more ways than his drug problems.

Imagine House having an awakening – imagine a family member racing in with "Doctor, I found this – what do you think?"and skeptical House looking, discovering it made sense, and having an epiphany: patients might indeed help.

Imagine, then, a future episode where the young docs are stumped. Imagine that House turns to them, pivoting on his cane, and sneers, "Okay, you're out of answers; have you asked the family if they found anything??"

That's the future of medicine.

4.

Let patients help
with quality and safety

This is a sensitive subject, because to a large extent most of us are in denial about it. (The Appendix will talk about this.) Thousands of people die every day from medical errors, but that's unthinkable to most of us, because most patients *don't* die.

I've never met anyone who doesn't want to fix this, but I've met plenty who don't want to *talk* about it. That makes it hard to improve. We could do two things about this: we could pound on clinicians to bear all the burden, or we can let patients help:

- **When the patient or family asks to look at the chart,** make it available: most charts contain errors. Remember, this data *will* get read sometime; the only reason to record information (on paper or in a computer) is so someone can read it back later. Why not let the family proofread?
- **When the patient or family wants to check the meds** that are being given, welcome it.
- **When they say, "I didn't see you wash your hands,"** thank them and do it.

And so on – you get the picture.

This isn't just a patients' rights issue. Of course patients have the most at stake in a medical error, but it's also a disservice to any clinician to make them work in a dangerous setting and bear the crushing burden when something goes wrong. It broke my heart to hear of the pediatric nurse in Seattle who *killed herself* in 2011[1] after a child in her care died from an error. Imagine how bad she must have felt, to end her life leaving three children of her own behind.

The unpleasant truth is that these people – with all their years of training – pretty much work without a net, without the safeguards we think are normal in other parts of life. Our streets have curbs to protect against driving on sidewalks; a diesel hose won't fit in your gas tank; yet even though hospitals are deadly places, protections like that commonly don't exist.

We can stay in denial and pray (literally) things will go well. But we can also wake up and be truthful with each other. Providers, we need a safer medical workplace. But until we have it, *let patients help*. The heart you save from breaking may be your own.

Let patients help… prevent preventable disasters.

Let patients help… prevent preventable lawsuits.

---

[1] http://well.blogs.nytimes.com/2011/07/06/when-nurses-make-mistakes/ (Search for "When Nurses Make Mistakes")

5.

Let patients help
control the cost of care

Some people won't like this chapter because they benefit from high medical spending. Everyone else, saddle up:

> To reduce spending, simply let patients know what everything will cost, and let them know they have options. Watch what happens.

In 2012 the Institute of Medicine said there's $750 billion of unnecessary spending in American medicine. That's a lot of money, and the people who receive it aren't eager for the flow to stop.[1] For instance, when I chose high-deductible insurance[2] in 2011, bills that used to fly past me (to be paid by insurance) stopped at my mailbox. They made no sense, and as I tried to shop for options, I learned it can be really hard to find out what spending is necessary and what's not.

It was eye-opening, and ultimately empowering. It woke me up.

---

[1] In 2006 the brilliant health economist Uwe Reinhardt published an article titled "Hospital pricing in America: Chaos behind a veil of secrecy." I'm not making this up; google it. And you wonder why costs keep rising? See also Stephen Brill's 25,000 word exposé – bigger than this book! – "Bitter Pill: Why medical bills are killing us" on the cover of *Time*, March 4, 2013.

[2] "High deductible" means you pay a lot of the bills yourself before insurance pays anything.

First I got an EOB[1] for a CAT scan:[2] $1,736, straight out of my pocket. Fifteen line items were listed, with no explanation. I called and asked, "What are all these things?" My insurance company said, "We don't know." I said, "How can we tell if I was charged in error, or there was fraud?" And I was told, "Oh, if there were fraud we'd do something about it."

From that moment on I behaved like an ordinary consumer – and it turns out I'm a lot better shopper than my insurance company. I'd ask them "How much should this vaccine cost?" and they'd say, "We don't know." I asked "How much should this skin cancer cost," and they said "We don't have that information. Ask your hospital." The hospital said, "We don't know – it depends on your insurance."

And yet in 2012 at the big TEDMED conference at the Kennedy Center in Washington, a speaker from Quest Diagnostics gave a talk on why "patients make lousy consumers." Really, Quest? Try giving us some facts, and then we'll see who can shop. (*Your lab* was one of the providers who said "We don't know.")

For my skin cancer I decided to do the grunt work myself and ask, ask, ask until I got answers. Everyone I spoke to was courteous, but they didn't have the information! I called three different hospitals, and every time they had to go digging. They were helpful, *but they had no experience* at answering "What will this cost?" But this will change as patients start to ask.

If you're a bulldog of a shopper – or know someone who is – you can do what I did: sink your teeth into this question and don't let go. After all, patients are the ultimate stakeholder – give *patients* price lists, and data on quality and safety.

Then we can get to the next step:

---

[1] EOB: Explanation of Benefits – the usually-cryptic sheet of codes and numbers you get from your insurance company, supposedly explaining all the good things they did for you. I once blogged that the Federal Trade Commission should ban calling something an "explanation" if nobody can understand it. Can you understand yours? Have you complained?

[2] For more on these efforts, search "cost-cutting" on epatientdave.com.

Let Patients Help!

6.

Let patients vote on what's worth the cost

This brings us to a deeper question: if we want to improve value in medical spending, who gets to say what value is in the first place?

Is it anything a doctor says is best for you? If so, what if different doctors disagree? (They usually do.)

Is it whichever treatment has the best-looking data? If so, is the data measuring what's important to *you*? I know a mom whose baby had persistent seizures. A major children's hospital told the family they had to switch to a new treatment, but other parents said the new way made life miserable. Who gets to say what's important?

The hospital was paternalistic: they said *they* knew, and the family's opinion was worth nothing. They made them go to another hospital.

Do you feel that's right? Some people feel it's the professional's duty to insist on following the best numbers – but what if there *aren't* any measurements for what the family cares about, because the researchers didn't ask what patients want studied? (They rarely do – because scientists usually consider it their job to know what's important.)

Should we spend more on cures, or more on prevention? Which is more valuable? Patients with chronic conditions often want *relief* more than they want more scientific understanding of *why* it hurts.

This will be vitally important as we curtail excess spending, as the Institute of Medicine says we must. People in the industry will naturally fight to preserve their jobs. That's fine with me, but we *must* be sure that as cuts are made, **families' wants are heard** loud and clear, or families will surely be steamrollered. Let patients help set priorities.

7.

Let patients use
their informed shopper skills

The business world has been transformed by consumerism: the ability of shoppers to size up their options, choose what they want, and reward the ones they like. That hasn't yet come to American medicine: families are barely starting to have comparison shopping tools.

This isn't just a "patients' rights" issue – if the best providers aren't publicly known, how can the market reward them? Let *informed* patients help improve medicine.

Patient as fiscal scapegoat

As I mentioned earlier, at the big TEDMED conference, an industry speaker said, "Patients make lousy consumers." Really?? Let's go to definitions: empowered consumers are people who...

- decide what they want
- research their options (for price, quality, convenience and service / satisfaction)
- make an informed choice.

Can you do that in medicine?

If you're told you need to have Treatment X done, can *you* find out:

- Who-all in your area does that procedure?

- Good out-of-area options? (How far away is the best of those?)
- **Price:** Can you find out what the cost will be, both total cost and your out of pocket cost after insurance?
    - o Websites like Healthcare Blue Book and Castlight Health offer shopping tools through employers, but not to the public. Clear Health Costs is a new company whose data is open.
- **Quality:**
    - o *Positive (success rates):* to my knowledge there's no published information anywhere on how often a particular hospital succeeds at a given treatment.
    - o *Negative (complications):* Websites like Hospital Compare and Leapfrog Group's Hospital Safety Scores publish infection rates and overall death rates from accidents and complications. In the safest hospitals in America, 5% of their surgical patients die later from complications. But there's no way (yet) to get that information for individual procedures.
- **Convenience** is simpler – location and hours. But some offer more: online appointment scheduling, online medical records and online bill payment can make a big difference in the overall customer experience.
- **Service and satisfaction:** We don't yet have good information on whose patients are happiest, but the government's "HCAHPS" scores are a step in the right direction, and doctor rating sites like HealthGrades are a start.

When patients have *that* kind of data, *then* we'll see if they're good consumers. Until then, it's abusive to insult them.

One final culture note: Have you ever asked a hospital or doctor what their infection rate is? Most people can't imagine asking. But this too will change – and the best providers will *advertise* their answers.

Consumerism works. But only when we know our options.

8.
Let patients help
make treatment decisions

The proper practice of medicine is moving from informed **consent** ("here's what I'll do – sign here to consent") to informed **choice** ("there are several options, with pros and cons. Let's discuss before you choose.") You have every right to be told about options for any decision; you have every right to ask.

During my fateful physical in 2006, Dr. Sands told me that at age 56 I should start thinking about prostate testing. He said *think about it -* he didn't say to do it.

He said, "The thing is, there's no test that says definitively whether there's a problem, and even if there is, it's not clear what to do about it, because there's no treatment that's best for everyone. A false positive can actually *cause* problems, getting treated for something that's not there."

Years later I learned that he had exemplified how doctors should approach this topic with men. The truth is that prostate treatment options often have important side effects, including incontinence (wearing a diaper the rest of your life) and impotence.[1] And decades

---

[1] Uncertain medical issues take on real impact if you apply the questions to issues in your undies.

of research have shown that even the best-intentioned physicians are lousy at guessing what a given patient wants.

The remedy is so simple: explain it to the patient, and let him decide. It's called Shared Decision Making – SDM. Founded by Dr. Jack Wennberg in the 1970s, the field now has decades of research fortifying its methods and benefits.

Yet even this isn't automatically simple: if a patient is to be empowered and enabled, they must *get* the message. And too often the choices aren't explained well.[1]

I'm not kidding – this matters. In 2012 I had the thrill of sharing a keynote with Dr. Wennberg, and he said that after years of trying, "Ultimately it came down to peeing better or sex. And when we put it those terms, shared decision making *flowed* into the conversation."

Clarity is power. Indeed.

---

[1] Tip for providers: try the "teachback" method – ask the patient to repeat back what you just told them. Tip for patients: if you're not asked to "teach back," ask to do it! Say, "Could I repeat that back, to see if I understood it?" And if the doc doesn't have time, call a nurse later.

Let Patients Help!

9.

Let patients help set research priorities

This subject's deeper, but when someone you love has an incurable disease it sure hits home. And highly engaged patient communities have some pretty strong feelings.

The purpose of science – the scientific method – is to converge on reliable knowledge, so treatments and more research can be built on a solid foundation. But who gets to say how that's done? And who gets to say *what* research goals should be pursued?

If the disease is progressive, causing an inexorable decline … if your body is going, or your mind, what do you want researchers to seek? Do you want:

- Deeper understanding of **why it's happening?** This is **science**, straight-up – the pursuit of knowledge.

- **Symptom relief**, even if we don't know why it works? This is more like **engineering**.

- **A wider range** of potential treatments? That's what happens when there's a race for **innovation.**

Knowing why it happens may someday lead to a more certain cure. But, you may be dead. On the other hand, someday it might help your descendants. Who gets to set the priority?

My Parkinson's friends feel strongly about this. My friends with Rheumatoid Disease feel so strongly that they renamed the condition from "rheumatoid arthritis" – based on *evidence* that science had named it wrong. Now they're defining their own research agenda. Should science listen, or hole up?

This isn't anti-science, it's *partnership* with science. Both the Parkinson's Pipeline Project and Rheumatoid Patient Foundation have rigorous standards and are respected by scientists. The questions they come up with seem endless and valid:

- **What should research focus on** – better treatments, or prevention and cure? Who gets to say?

- **Who sets the bar on when to release new treatments,** and when to hold back because we're not sure enough if they're safe and effective?[1] My Parkinson's friend Perry said earlier, "Until your days are numbered, you don't *know* what's important."

- **What if something unexpected and good happens** during a trial? It's happened several times during Parkinson's studies, but researchers have rejected the unexpected good news, calling such placebo effect "noise" (not useful information), even cancelling some studies. But some placebo benefits have lasted *years after* the study stopped. Should science investigate why?? Patients sure think so: "Whatever that was, let's have more of it! Study it!"

In industry, if something useful happened by accident you *bet* the lab would pursue it. That's how Post-It notes were invented (a failed adhesive – it wouldn't stay stuck), and it's even how Viagra's magic effect was discovered: it was a cardiac drug, but some patients reported a rousing side effect.

Who gets to say where research money should be spent?

---

[1] The AIDS/HIV movement objected loudly and successfully to the establishment's priorities. Is this different from other progressive diseases?

10.

Let patients say
what patient-centered means

In the years ahead this will be an increasing imperative. The business of medicine must be much more patient centered. But to someone who's always thought from the institution's point of view, that's hard to do.

My friend Cristin Lind has a new litmus test for whether a clinic is patient-centered: when they give you an appointment time, is it the time *you* have to be there, or the time *the clinician* will see you?

- The patient-centered view is "I have to be there at 8:30"
- The clinic-centered view is "Our resource [the clinician, the scanner, etc.] is booked at 8:40."

See? Patient-centered is from the patient's view; anything else is not.

My own hospital was the same: before my 3 pm CT scan, I'd have to arrive much earlier to drink the magic goop that lets them see my innards. In *my* calendar I had to write 1:30, but on their patient portal all I saw was when *their asset* (the scanner) was booked: 3 pm.

Then, for the follow-up meeting with the care team, the portal said I had three appointments, all at the same time! Turns out it was *one* appointment in my calendar – but three of *their* resources were involved. Three clinicians, in the same room at the same time.

Patient-centered view: one appointment. Business-centered view: three appointments.

Forward-thinking hospitals are already changing this, and I have a prediction: in the coming years, some practices and some hospitals will start acting like customer-centered businesses – and the ones who don't will start to look disorganized and rude. And that will shake the confidence of any consumer.

Fortunately, the remedy is truly simple: just listen, *really listen*, to what your patient-customers are trying to tell you. To hear it you may need to give up your own point of view.

In short, let patients help make your business more competitive.

Part 3: Tip sheets:

How To Be e-Patients and Empowering Providers

Including Dr. Danny Sands' guide to
safe, effective web use

Ten things e-patients say to engage in their care

> ## 1. The magic incantation
> *Say this one, and boom: you're being engaged:*
>
> **"I'm the kind of person who likes to understand as much as I can about my health. Can I ask some questions?"**

2. "I found this site. What do you think?"

3. "How can I talk with other patients?" (Online or off)

4. "What will this cost?"
   At this writing, hardly anyone knows. Help change that: keep asking.

5. "Are there any other options?"
   "What happens if I choose 'do nothing'?"

6. "How strong is the evidence?"

7. "What's your infection rate?"

8. "Could I see my chart?"
   [or my mother's / my child's / my friend's, if you're authorized]

9. "This isn't right in the chart / didn't happen / is missing. Please fix it."

10. "What's the standard of care for my condition? When was it updated?"

Ten things clinicians say
that encourage patient engagement

By Dr. Danny Sands

1. "I'm here to work together with you on your health. We are a team."

2. "Learn as much as you can about your condition. Here are some ways to get started."

3. "Talk about your condition with other patients like you."

4. "I encourage you to seek a second opinion before making a decision about major surgery or other serious treatments."

5. "I don't know the answer to your question; let's look it up together."

6. "There are a number of options, each with pros and cons. Let's talk about your preference."

7. "Here's how you can connect with me online."

8. "Here are the things I'd like to address today; what are your concerns?"

9. "Did I address all of your concerns? Is there anything else?"

10. "Feel free to read your test results and the rest of your medical record online whenever you wish. You can also use our website to schedule an appointment, request a prescription renewal, or do other administrative tasks."

Ten things clinicians say (or do) that <u>dis</u>courage patient engagement

By Dr. Danny Sands

1. "Here's what you're going to do."

2. "Stay off the internet. If you do search, don't bring it to us—we don't have time for it."

3. "We'll call you if anything's wrong. If you want to get your test results, you'll need to make an appointment."

4. "If you want to see your medical record, talk to the office – they'll tell you the fee."

5. "Don't try to diagnose and treat yourself—I'm the doctor."

6. "I know our phones are always busy, but that's the only way to reach us."

7. *Usually thought but not said:* "I'm not happy you sought a second opinion; don't you trust me?"

8. Dictating the visit agenda without asking for patient input

9. "We've done everything I needed to do today. Sorry we haven't got time for your issues. Please make another appointment."

10. Not calling patients back—making them come in to the office instead.

Let Patients Help!

For patients: collaborating effectively with your clinicians

By Dr. Danny Sands
(and approved by e-Patient Dave!)

1. Appreciate that healthcare should be a collaboration among the patient, the patient's caregivers and family, and clinicians.

2. Be mutually respectful of each other's contributions. Your physician is an expert in medicine, but you are an expert in you.

3. Take responsibility for your health—healthcare is not a spectator sport: it's participatory.

4. Prepare for your visit: read about your conditions, review your record, make a list so you don't forget, and discuss the agenda in advance.

5. Understand that you're not your doctor's only patient, so respect her time. If some issues really can wait, perhaps another appointment is appropriate. Be respectful of time in your online communication, as well—don't try to manage something in e-mail that your doctor may be more comfortable discussing on the phone or in an appointment.

6. Communicate—and if your doctor can't, either speaking or listening, find one who can. If the communication fails, you're the one who suffers most.

7. Take notes, and get copies of your clinician's.

8. Don't demand tests or treatments from your physician—discuss them. Your doctor may have good reasons for saying yes, or no; be a good partner.

9. Be responsible for your wellbeing. Keep in touch. Do your part, do what you can to care for yourself, and get professional help when needed.

10. Give your care team constructive feedback, both good and bad. Listen to what you hear back, and accept feedback on your own participation. That's partnership.

Dr. Danny Sands' rules for smart web use

There's a wealth of online health information, most of which is of good quality and is available free. But amid the gold there's also garbage: it may be bad information or may be biased, sometimes because the author is peddling something or may have a fixed false belief, or because of commercial sponsorship with no clear editorial guidelines that create a clear dividing line between sponsorship and medical content.

Follow some simple rules to avoid being led astray or injuring yourself:

1. Ask your doctor if she has any suggestions on where to start looking—she may know of some useful sites.

2. Learn how to identify good vs. bad health websites, using guidelines such as:
    a. MLANet – the Medical Library Association's website.[1] See their *MLA User's Guide to Finding and Evaluating Health Information on the Web* and *Deciphering Medspeak*
    b. MedlinePlus Videos and Cool Tools.[2] See the buttons *Evaluating Health Information* and *Understanding Medical Words*
    c. The code of conduct at Health on the Net[3]

3. Other patients can often direct you to useful websites, as well. But just because they are recommended by a peer does not automatically make them reliable—apply the filtering criteria above to these websites, as well.

4. Don't take an online diagnosis too seriously until confirmed by a healthcare professional. It may be accurate, but it could make

---

[1] MLAnet.org/resources/consumr_index.html
[2] nlm.nih.gov/medlineplus/videosandcooltools.html
[3] HON.ch/HONcode/Patients/Conduct.html

you worry about something much more serious than you have (or the other way around). Especially avoid online diagnosis if you have a tendency to be anxious.

5. Government Departments of Health often have excellent online health resources. In the US, this is MedlinePlus.gov. Some health provider systems do, as well, such as Kaiser, the Veterans Administration, and Mayo Clinic.

6. Clinical trials sites, such as ClinicalTrials.gov and others can be useful if you have a serious condition.

7. Don't be surprised to find that many articles you read are the same on different websites—many websites license articles from the same handful of sources.

8. Let your doctor know about websites you find useful—she may want to look at them and refer other patients to them.

9. Your doctor may have access to more detailed online resources that require a subscription, and may be able to give you temporary access or copies, sometimes with versions for patients or professionals. Ask for whichever you're more comfortable reading.

10. Use Google Scholar (scholar.google.com) or the National Library of Medicine's PubMed (pubmed.gov) if you want to find scientific papers on a particular topic.[1] Remember as you're doing this that just because a paper appears in a journal (even one claiming to be peer-reviewed) does not automatically mean it is good scholarship. Some journals have higher standards than others (and some obscure journals seems to have very low standards, indeed).

---

[1] In many cases, you'll only be able to read the abstract (a brief summary) for free—publishers can charge a ridiculous amount of money for access to single articles. However, you may be able to get full-text access to some of these papers for free through your hospital, local medical school library, or even by asking your doctor (but request these judiciously, because it is an inconvenience).

Ten things insurers & employers say to let patients help

This section is in beta! Submit your suggestions in comments on the Book page on epatientdave.com.

Employers, insurers, what do you do?
Patients, what do you want to hear from them?

1. "Here's how to be an e-patient – ten things e-patients say."

2. "Here are some providers who welcome engaged patients."

3. "Be engaged in your health. We cover prevention and check-ups 100%."

4. "We're putting a clinic in your workplace to make check-ups easy. Take advantage of it!"

5. "Here's what this should cost. And here are some tools to shop around, if you want."

6. "Know your standard of care. Here's how."

7. "Here are the facts on quality and safety for the doctors and hospitals in your area."

8. ?

9. ?

10. ?

Submit your suggestions!

Epilog:
The Road Ahead

As the first edition of this book goes to press, the role of the patient in health and care is changing fast. As I type these words the big health policy journal *Health Affairs* has just published an entire issue (February 2013) titled "New Era of Patient Engagement." It cites growing research that engaged patients do better and cost less. And if that isn't value, I don't know what is.

But the journal also makes clear that we have much to learn about how to do it successfully. This is the question that fascinates me in my work today, and it's a question in which the readers of this book will immerse themselves. We're creating a new culture.

Regardless of what happens at the policy level, culture change is real only when it alters **what people say to each other.** And that's where you come in. Yes, you, whether you're a patient yet, a provider, or anyone else in the world. You. What *you* say.

In this short book I've distilled my view of the movement into short sets of ten points and ten actions, with an even simpler title: Let Patients Help. Why short and simple? Because big books don't get read, but concise instructions are easy to grasp. And I want you to grasp these points.

Medicine could learn a lot from that.

Be a leader in your circle of friends and colleagues: speak differently.

About the Authors

"e-Patient Dave" deBronkart is a leading spokesperson for the patient engagement movement.

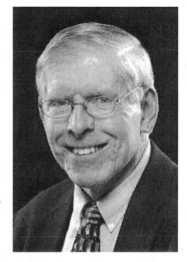

A highly rated international keynote speaker and policy advisor, he blogs at the Forbes "Let Patients Help" blog and his own site, ePatientDave.com. The "about" page on his website has more details.

Dr. Danny Sands, Dave's primary care physician, is passionate about healthcare transformation. A practicing physician with training and experience in clinical informatics, he has worked in a variety of capacities in the health care IT industry since 2004. In almost 14 years at Beth Israel Deaconess Medical Center he developed and implemented innovative systems to improve clinical care delivery and patient engagement, including clinical decision support systems, an electronic health record, and one of the nation's first patient portals.

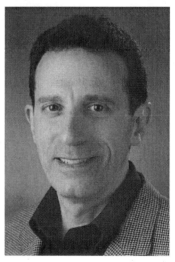

Dr. Sands is the recipient of numerous healthcare honors, including recognition in 2009 by *HealthLeaders* Magazine as one of "20 People Who Make Healthcare Better" (with Dave). He holds an academic appointment at Harvard Medical School and for twenty years has maintained a primary care practice in which he makes extensive use of health IT – much of which he helped to introduce during his tenure at Beth Israel Deaconess Medical Center.

Appendix:
Stop the denial.

Nobody wants to talk about this, but here it is:

Medicine can be dangerous, and clinicians work without a net.

One of the most painful truths for me to accept has been the rate of medical accidents and their horrible human cost, both to the patients and families involved and to the clinicians involved. Almost every corner of our medical culture fails to deal honestly with this; it's massive denial, which renders us impotent to solve it and makes every failure surprising, shocking, and painful.

Please, everyone, realize: **it's risky to cut someone open** (otherwise known as surgery), and **it can be risky to put potent chemicals in you** (aka medications.) Germs are everywhere and they get into cuts, and bodies are complex and variable: things go wrong.

Did you know that in the *best* hospitals in America, 1 in 20 surgical patients *dies of a complication*? *After* the surgery?[1] (In the worst hospitals it's 1 in 6.) Hard to believe, yes?

If you were considering surgery, wouldn't that change your thinking? Wouldn't it make "Let's wait a bit" seem like a prudent thought?

---

[1] See HospitalSafetyScores.org

You'll probably be told the risks specific to the surgery you'll get, but did they tell you the *overall* rate of deaths from complications at this hospital? (You do want to know, right? Actually many people don't.)

Wouldn't you like to know which hospitals are best? When you move to a new town, wouldn't you like to see Hospital Safety Scores on the map, along with school scores and the nearest fire stations?

The tough thing is, we can't solve this just by beating on providers, because **not all errors are caused by carelessness.** (Some errors are, but it's a giant mistake to assume they all are.) **Medicine is complicated and our systems are not fail-safe.**

Everyone who studies medicine knows the classic 1999 report *To Err is Human* that estimated up to 98,000 deaths a year in America from medical errors – 15 people every hour – and the number doubles when you include deaths from hospital acquired infections.[1] But not so many people know that a 2010 Medicare audit[2] showed **15%** of Medicare patients who went into a hospital were harmed, contributing to 15,000 Medicare deaths a month. 500 deaths a day!

That's deaths from complications, not from the disease.

This is a mixture of two toxic factors. First, clinician performance is no more perfect than patient performance: **both patients and providers stick to a plan about half the time:**

- Infections happen when germs move from patient to patient, often on clinicians' hands, clothes and equipment. Yet on average providers **wash hands between patients half the time.** (When you're in a hospital, as a patient or visitor, insist on it!)

---

[1] "Hospital acquired infection" (HAI) may just sound like a bad owie, but it's gruesome: these are infections that took over patients' bodies and *killed them.* My friend Pat Mastors, author of *Design to Survive*, had the horrible experience of watching her father suffer for six months, when the bacteria called *C. diff.* ran rampant in his gut and exploded his intestines. He died. That was after a simple knee replacement.

[2] oig.hhs.gov/oei/reports/oei-06-09-00090.pdf

- Doctors only **prescribe the standard of care**[1] about half the time,[2] for instance prescribing a baby aspirin for certain cardiac patients, inspecting the feet of a patient with diabetes, etc.

The other factor is that **clinicians work without a net:** unlike many workplaces, **hospitals don't have built-in safety measures** to prevent simple human error.

- In 2007 Dennis Quaid's two week old twins were accidentally given 1000 times too much blood thinner and started bleeding to death internally. (Amazingly, they were saved.) Analysis revealed that the correct bottle and the wrong bottle looked almost identical, *and* they were stored in the same part of the medication rack: it was way too easy to grab the wrong one without realizing it.

- Recall from the chapter "Let patients help take care of their families" the story of Duane Smith, who was saved miraculously after a head-on car crash, but later lost his fingers and toes. The care team was brilliant but they don't have a fail-safe workflow to make sure *everything* gets done.

Improvements are happening, but the error rates are real. Sometimes a common sense fix from other industries can help. I'm told anesthesia errors were greatly reduced when the hoses for different gases hoses were made to be different sizes, so you can no longer pump the wrong gas into the wrong hose. In other areas of life such physical safeguards are normal: you can't plug a 220 volt clothes dryer into a 110 volt outlet, and in gas stations the diesel and gas pumps are not interchangeable. But in medicine such protections are often absent.

---

[1] "Standard of care" is the standard things clinicians are supposed to do for a patient with certain conditions. Patients with a certain cardiac status should always be prescribed a baby aspirin every day; people with diabetes should always have their feet examined on every visit; things like that.

[2] Peter Margolis, Cincinnati Children's Hospital. Reported by Susannah Fox.

Our denial about these risks is costly. Not only does denial make us forget to be as careful as we should (and could!), but when something goes wrong, it can create a crushing burden on the professional who made the mistake. Remember, from "Let patients help with quality and safety," the pediatric nurse who killed herself after an error.

Imagine the remorse that must have filled her to take that step. It's simply a mistake to think that the cause of all errors is heartlessness. Fixing that, where it exists, won't make the problem go away.

This is not to say some professionals aren't responsible for mistakes. Sometimes there are. But it's just as big a mistake to assume that all errors are negligence. Good people can get hurt – on both sides.

What to do: Stop being in denial about the hazards, and the need for human caution. Clinicians and patients alike, get real:

- **Patients (and families)**
    - **Don't expect perfection.** Do expect *caution* and *carefulness*, including hand washing, every single time.
    - **Ask about the care plan,** so you can help follow along. Be involved – educate yourself, as much as you're able.
    - **Realize your clinicians may be in denial** about risks, which is dangerous. Help keep things on track.
    - **Double check** such things as whether the correct medication is being delivered.
    - **Ask to check the chart.**
    - **Ask what you can help keep an eye on.**

- **Clinicians**
    - **Don't act like there are no risks.**
    - **Be careful.** Wash hands, and encourage your peers to. Peer support is patient-centered, not rude.
    - **Let patients help.** When patients ask how they can help ensure safety, welcome the offer.

When accidents do happen:

I recommend the services of a Boston-based non-profit, MITSS: Medically Induced Trauma Support Services (mitss.org). Founded by Linda Kenney, victim of an accident that almost killed her, it's an inspiring organization that helps patients, families, and clinicians recover emotionally and move on with life.

MITSS has developed a toolkit that's been downloaded in 77 countries: *Tools for Building a Clinician and Staff Support Program.* It's for organizations to use regardless of where they are on the spectrum – from those in the early stages of looking at different support models to those who may already have programs in place. To download it, search "toolkit" at MITSStools.org.

MITSS is a great example of what can happen when we ... let patients help.

Even in the worst of circumstances.

What ways have you seen where patients have helped, or could help?

What ways have you seen where patients have helped, or could help?

What ways have you seen where patients have helped, or could help?

What ways have you seen where patients have helped, or could help?

What ways have you seen where patients have helped, or could help?

What ways have you seen where patients have helped, or could help?

What ways have you seen where patients have helped, or could help?

What ways have you seen where patients have helped, or could help?

What ways have you seen where patients have helped, or could help?

What ways have you seen where patients have helped, or could help?

What ways have you seen where patients have helped, or could help?